CONTENTS

DEDICATION	4
Preface to the Readers	5
Preface to the Parents and Educators	6
Chapter 1 - Freddy's New Nest	7
Chapter 2 - Tommy, the Terrifying Tomcat	13
Chapter 3 - The Delicious French Fries	17
Chapter 4 - Freddy's Nightmare	21
Chapter 5 - Freddy Can't Fly	26
Chapter 6 - Working Hard	32
Chapter 7 - Time to Exercise!	34
Chapter 8 - Freddy Has a Rest	39
Chapter 9 - The Hawk	42
Chapter 10 - Safe and Sound	47
Testimonials	51

Dedication

To sincere Friends and strong Friendships

Acknowledgment

Thank you to all who have worked on this book. It has been a fascinating and fun journey.

DiDi

Freddy's French Fries Fiasco

By DiDi LeMay

A Flair For Writing-Publishing Services

Copyright © 2012 by DiDi LeMay

ALL RIGHTS RESERVED.

This book contains material protected under International and Federal Copyright Laws and Treaties. Any unauthorized reprint or use of this material is prohibited. No part of this book may be reproduced or transmitted in any form or by any means, electronic or mechanical, including photocopying, recording, or by any information storage and retrieval system without express written permission from the author/publisher.

A Flair For Writing-Publishing Services

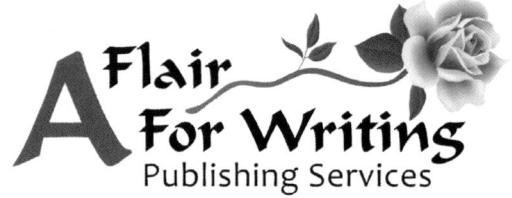

First Edition, August 2012
First Printing, August 2012

Edited by Donna Erickson, Abington, MA
www.AFlairForWriting.com
Book Design: Charlie Davis, Northfield, MA
Cover Illustration: Charlie Davis, Northfield, MA
www.DavisImages.com
Inside Illustrations: Jacquie Campbell
Printed in the United States of America

ISBN 978-1-4675-2963-1
Library of Congress Control Number: 2012909495

To the Readers

This is not a story about french fries—or, chips, candy, ice cream, chocolate, or cake.

This is a story about Freddy, how he got too fat to fly, and how his friends supported him in his quest to lose weight and learn to fly again. His friends are important to him, and they encouraged him in his pursuit to become healthy.

I met Freddy, a young sparrow, on a warm summer afternoon in a beautiful park by the lake. He and his friends, Alfie, Jeanie, and Robby, were playing a game of tag. As they hopped, flew, and danced on the ground and in the air, I was amused as I watched their escapades, and my imagination started to wander. The little birds inspired me. I wanted to tell their story of friendship and camaraderie.

I saw there was one sparrow that was bigger than the other three. He reminded me of myself when I was young, a bit awkward and clumsy because of extra weight. I realized I wanted to share my own story of being overweight— especially how important it is to be healthy and how being healthy allows you to have more fun. I am very thankful to my friends who encouraged me on my mission to lose weight by doing exercises with me--convincing me that I did not need that piece of cake or ice cream cone and letting me know how proud of me they were.

While Freddy and his friends have their adventures, they learn about healthy eating. Friendships develop, and the experiences they have bring them closer together.

DiDi LeMay

Preface to Parents and Educators

The story of Freddy is near and dear to my heart. I understand his struggle with being overweight.

A few years ago, I was quite overweight. Some would have said I was obese. I finally decided enough is enough and started to learn about healthy eating and exercising. Bit by bit, I lost weight and ultimately achieved a total weight loss of more than one hundred pounds.

During the last few years, I have seen more and more children who are overweight. This concerns me greatly because of the possible consequences to their health and happiness.

I felt motivated to help them deal with the issue of childhood obesity because I also had experienced being overweight. I know how important it is to be healthy and how valuable friends are. Their support was vital during the time I was fighting "the battle of the bulge."

I wanted to share my experiences and help give them insight by showing them they can lose weight, be healthy, and have the support of their friends. I felt it was important to express that being healthy is fun because you can do more.

I wish, with all my heart, that Freddy and his friends—Alfie, Jeanie, and Robbie—are able to give kids the courage and determination to live full, happy, and healthy lives with many, many dear friends.

DiDi LeMay

Chapter 1

Freddy's New Nest

Amongst the gravel and windblown leaves, a young, chubby sparrow named Freddy stood back to check out his handiwork. With his wings on his hips and a big grin on his face, he sighed.

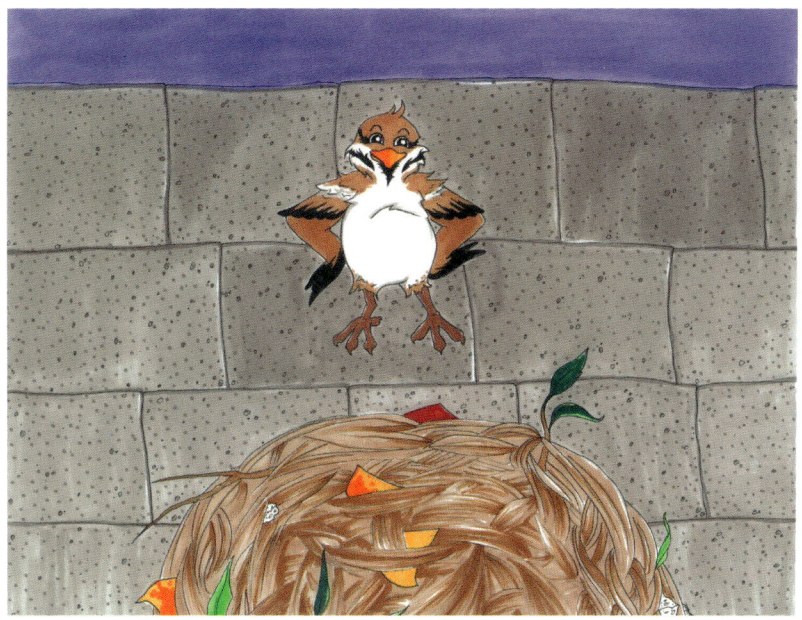

"Phew!" said Freddy as he wiped his forehead.

He had worked very hard to build a new nest. While flying here and there, he had gathered twigs and bits of grass. He had also collected pieces of greasy paper in colorful, funny-looking shapes. Freddy had stuffed the paper between the twigs and grass. Styrofoam helped cushion his nest and was very interesting to Freddy because it was thick, warm, and also, waterproof. All of those qualities were important to him. After all, his nest was his home!

Freddy felt proud of himself. This was the first time he had ever built a nest. His parents had given him permission to

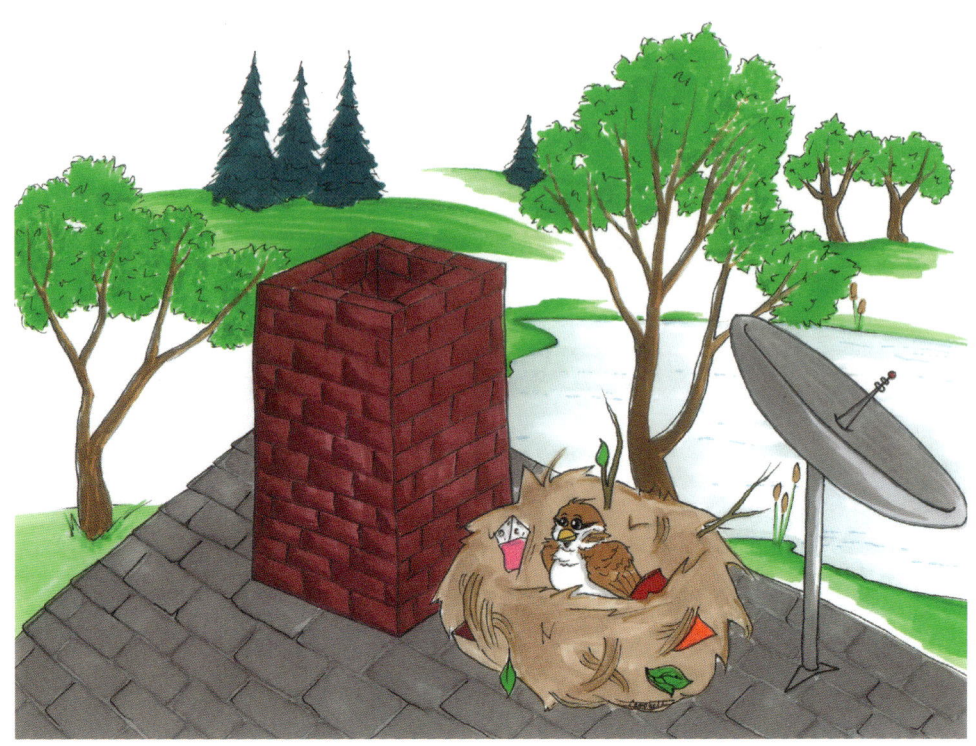

move from the family nest, in the tree nearby, to his own nest on the rooftop.

His new nest was hidden between the warm chimney of a restaurant and a small satellite dish with bits of old paint and flakes of rust. Freddy proudly paced back and forth on the rooftop. He was so clever! His new nest would keep him warm in the winter because the steam and smoke from the chimney flowed past it. Also, he would be able to smell the delicious aromas coming from the restaurant below—this always made him especially hungry.

Freddy settled into his new nest and squinted his eyes against the bright sunshine. He was curious and felt like a grown-up bird. He looked around and listened to all the sights and sounds nearby. To his left, he saw the trees where his parents lived, with treetops full of deep green leaves that rustled in the soft breeze. The lake shimmered as the sun shone brightly in the clear, blue sky. A few puffy, white clouds floated by lazily. In the distance, Freddy heard a few geese noisily arguing. He wondered what they were so angry about.

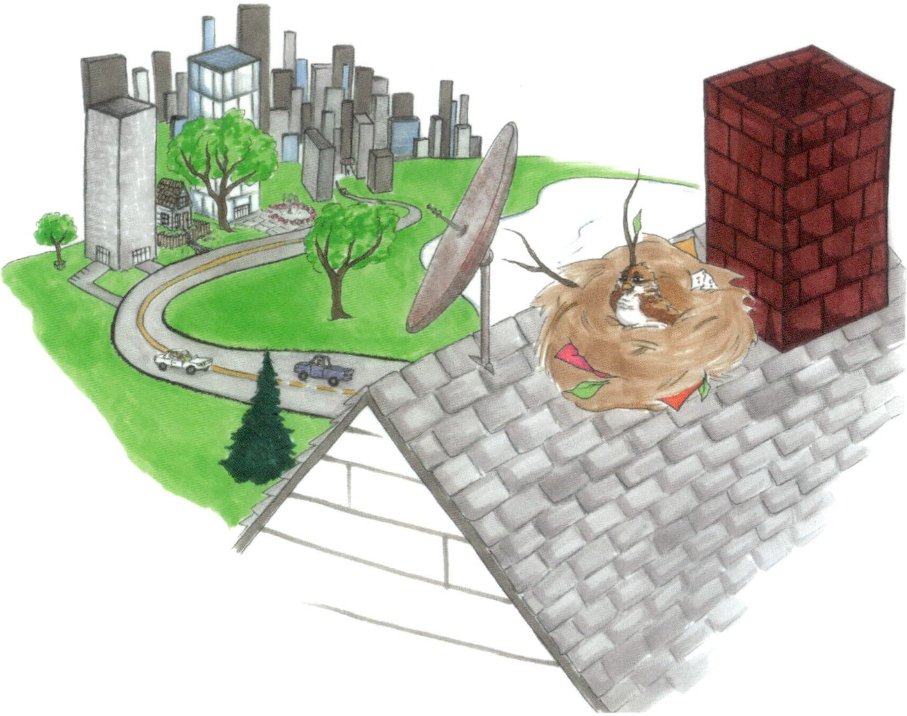

Turning and cocking his little feathered head to the right, he saw shiny cars humming along a grey ribbon of highway. He saw two tall buildings reaching up to the sky.

The sun reflected in the large windows, making them sparkle. The view was beautiful and very interesting. All the action, the cars driving on the road, the sun reflecting in the windows of the two tall buildings and the children running along the lake caught Freddy's attention. It was like watching action on TV.

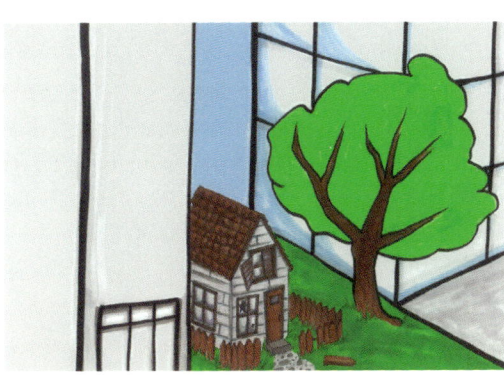

Snuggled between the two tall buildings was a small, run-down house with an overgrown yard. Freddy knew an old, grey tomcat lived in that house.

His name was Tommy, and he was always on the lookout to catch birds. Tommy's fur was matted, and he had old battle scars on his nose. His bright green eyes always glared.

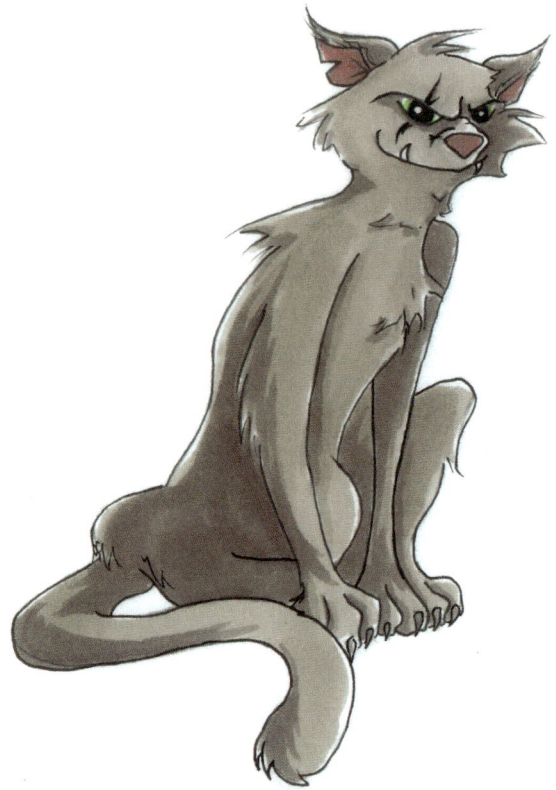

Tommy looked scary! He knew Freddy and his friends liked to fly around the yard, and Tommy would get excited because he wanted to catch them. Freddy's parents had warned him about the dangers of being in that backyard.

As it gradually turned dark, cars continued to drive along the road. Freddy noticed their pretty white and red lights. Sometimes lots of lights appeared, and other times there were not that many.

All day long, humans had come and gone. They had arrived at the restaurant in shiny cars and jumped out. Laughing and talking, they had run into the building. After a while, they had come out with arms full of colorful bags filled with food—very yummy food! Freddy had tried the food and found it very tasty! He smacked his yellow beak as he thought of the delicious food.

During the past few weeks, Freddy had met and interacted with a few little humans—children. He especially liked the children. They had given him lots of little yellow sticks—french fries, the children called them. The children had arrived with their mothers and fathers and sat outside to eat their food— the yummy french fries!

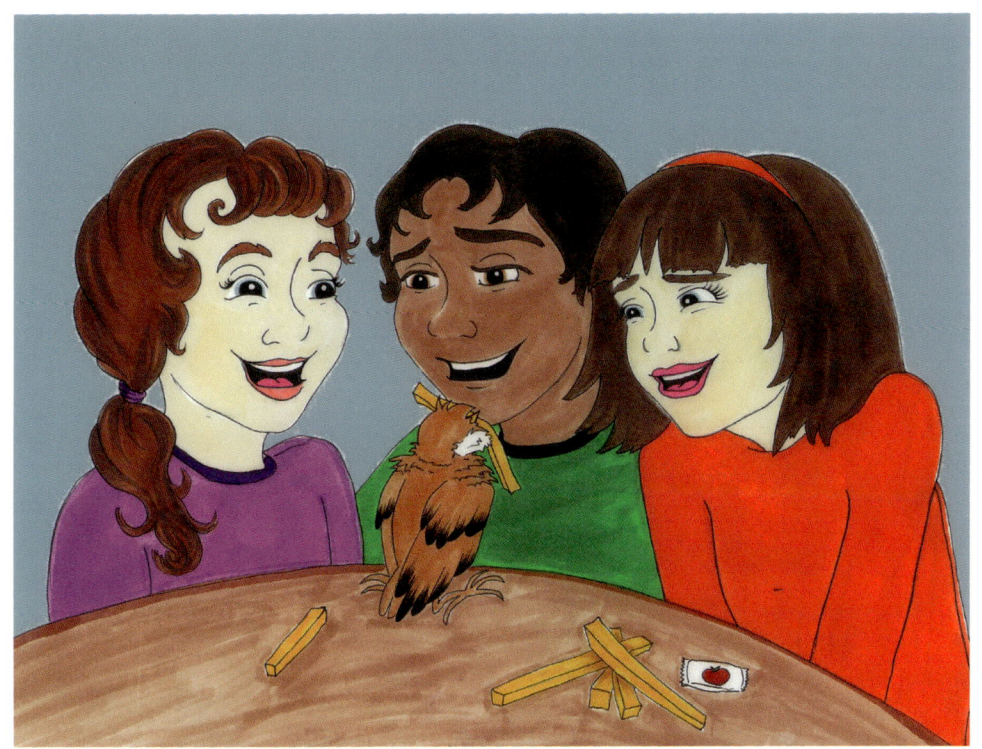

Today was a very lazy day for Freddy. He had just met a few humans, and they had fed him a lot of french fries. *Oh, they are so yummy!* thought Freddy as he fluttered his wings and smacked his little yellow beak.

A few minutes later, Freddy was lazily dozing off. *Hmm, this is so nice and quiet.* His little black head nodded and he was soon fast asleep in the warm, bright sunlight.

"Hey, Freddy! Hey!" called out a small brown bird. "Hey, come out and play with us!"

"Huh?" Freddy woke up with a start. "What... huh...what?"

"Freddy, over here. It's me, Alfie!" yelled the little brown bird waving his wings.

Alfie was excited and could not sit still. He hopped on his left leg, then his right leg, then on the left, and then on the right one again. His two little friends, Jeanie and Robby, were waiting for him in the nearest treetop where they lived with their parents.

"Jeanie, Robby, and I are going to play. We're all going to play together! We're going to fly over the lake!" squawked Alfie to no one in particular. "I'm so excited. We're going to catch some insects and spy on Tommy, the tomcat. We're even going to fly without flapping our wings. That is so dangerous! C'mon, Freddy, c'mon. It'll be so much fun!"

Freddy slowly stretched out his wings and yawned. "Nah, I don't feel like it. I'm tired. I want to take a nap."

Alfie shrugged his little shoulders, turned around, and yelled, "Robby! Jeanie! Let's go. Let's have some fun!"

Chapter 2
Tommy, the Terrifying Tomcat

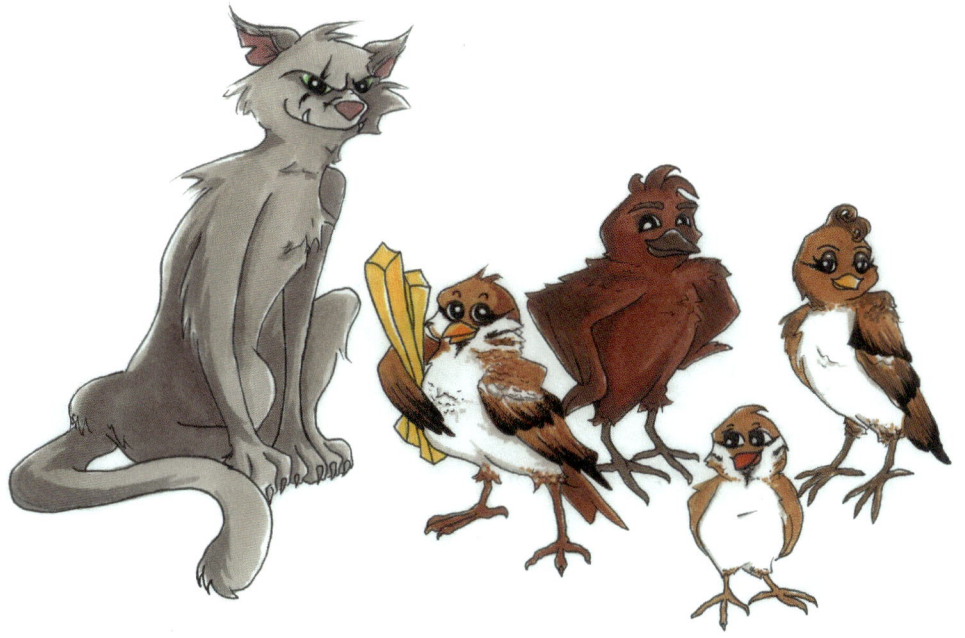

Alfie's two little friends took flight from the green treetop. The breeze stirred the dark green leaves causing a soft rustling sound. Side by side, the three little friends headed to the lake. A few ducks and swans glided through the water enjoying the warmth and quiet of an idle summer's day.

"Whoo-hoo!" yelled Jeanie as she swooped down to catch some small insects.

"Hey, Jeanie, look at me! I'm floating through the air. I'm not flapping my wings!" shouted Robby.

Giggling, Jeanie swooped down to catch up with him.

"Oh, Robby, you are such a show-off!" squealed Jeanie as she flapped her wings.

"Hey, guys," called Alfie. "Look. Tommy, the tomcat is sleeping! Let's go drink from his water bowl. It'll be a really exciting game!"

"Alfie, you know that's dangerous!" gasped Jeanie.

"That sounds like so much fun!" chuckled Robby.

"Oh Jeanie, it'll be fun! Let's go!" twittered Alfie.

Off the three friends went. Squawking and squealing while pretending to be dive-bombers, they headed directly towards the overgrown backyard where Tommy was lounging in a patch of sunlight.

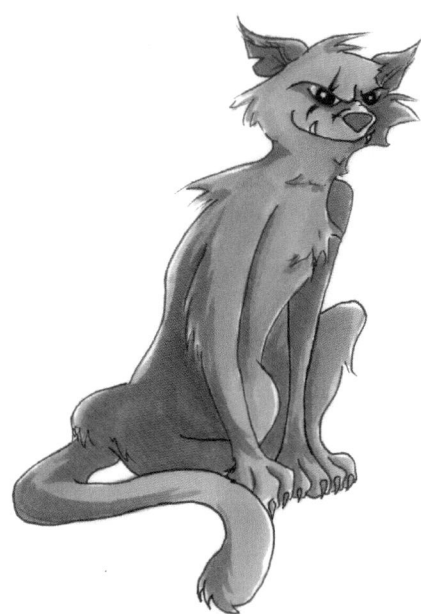

Hiding in the thorn bushes, the three friends waited. The breeze rustled the leaves, and the little sparrows swayed on a branch, waiting for just the right moment. They were so excited, they could hardly stay quiet. This was a very dangerous adventure and their eyes shone brightly with anticipation.

Tommy stretched and rolled onto his back. His front paws were spread out above his head. His head was rolled to one side and he had a peaceful grin on his ragged face. Once in a while he licked his lips, and the little sparrows could see that there were only a few teeth left in his mouth.

One by one, the little friends flew to the cracked ceramic bowl that stood next to an old, rusty garbage can. Alfie stood on the edge of the bowl and took a sip of water. Jeanie gasped. Alfie was so brave!

Next, Jeanie quietly swooped down and landed on the garbage can. She hopped to the edge and jumped toward the water bowl. She was just about to take a sip when Robby loudly crash-landed on top of the garbage can. The sound echoed through the quiet afternoon and woke up Tommy.

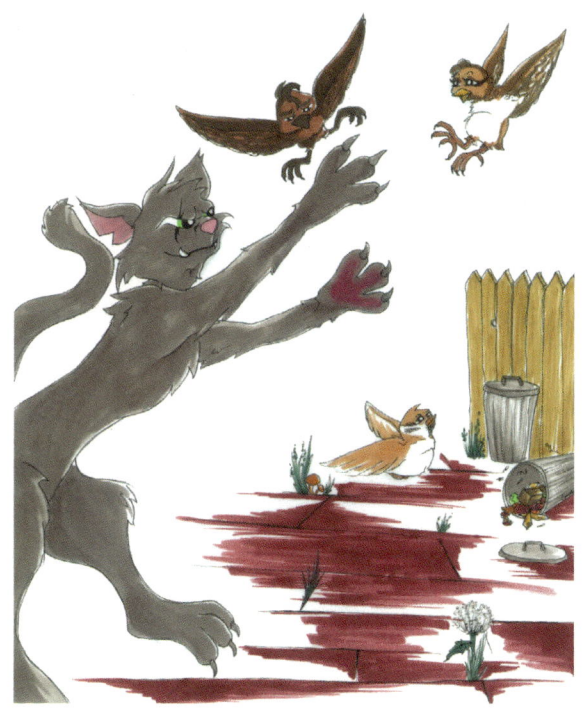

In one smooth move, Tommy jumped up and looked around. In an instant he saw the little sparrows and pounced towards them. His claws were facing the birds, and they glistened in the sunlight. They looked very big and sharp. His bright green eyes were mesmerizing as he glared at the little birds.

Alfie jumped up, flapped his wings, and off he went into the bushes. Jeanie quickly fluttered over to the nearest tree. But poor Robby looked around, dazed after his topsy-turvy landing.

Tommy saw Robby and quietly crouched down, getting ready to pounce. Just then, Alfie and Jeanie fluttered around Tommy. They needed to give Robby time to escape.

Tommy jumped up on his hind legs and swatted at them with his long front paws.

Robby got up and flew to safety, as Jeanie and Alfie followed close behind. Tommy didn't give up, though. He continued jumping and swatting while following them. Tommy began hissing and meowing, which made him look quite scary.

The birds finally reached the fence and landed on the other side. Their feathers were ruffled, and their little hearts were pounding inside their chests. They were panting so hard that their tiny chests were heaving, and they couldn't catch their breath. Their yellow beaks opened widely to get more air. With a panicked look on each of their tiny faces, the three friends huddled together.

Tommy's face was pushed against the fence.

"Next time I will get you!" hissed Tommy. "How dare you drink my water! That's my water. Get your own!" Tommy then turned around, walked away, and went to lie down in his favorite spot in the sun.

"Phew! That was close," panted Alfie.

"He was so mean!" chirped Jeanie.

"Let's do it again!" chimed Robby.

Alfie had lost interest. "Nah, I think we should go see Freddy."

Chapter 3

The Delicious French Fries

Freddy had just woken up from his nap. After stretching, yawning, and looking about, he saw his three friends being chased by Tommy, the tomcat who lived in the garden.

"Oh no!" called out Freddy as he anxiously watched Tommy chasing his friends.

When his friends finally reached the other side of the fence, Freddy relaxed.

I'm hungry again, and thirsty, too, thought Freddy. With a sigh, he struggled out of his nest made of Styrofoam, twigs, and paper. He waddled through the gravel and tar to the edge of the roof. Freddy then carefully peered over the edge to see if any of the children had left those wonderful yellow sticks—french fries. He also loved that yummy brown water they called *pop*.

While Freddy was peaking over the edge of the roof, he did not notice that his three friends were sneaking up behind him. Step by step, they quietly crept closer and closer until suddenly...

"Boo!" they yelled out in chorus.

With a yelp, Freddy jumped and nearly fell off the roof. He flapped his wings vigorously, so he would not topple to the ground below.

He turned to his friends. With a frown on his face, he yelled, "Hey, that's not nice!"

Alfie chuckled. He admitted he had been wrong to frighten Freddy. "Well, okay. What were you doing, anyway?"

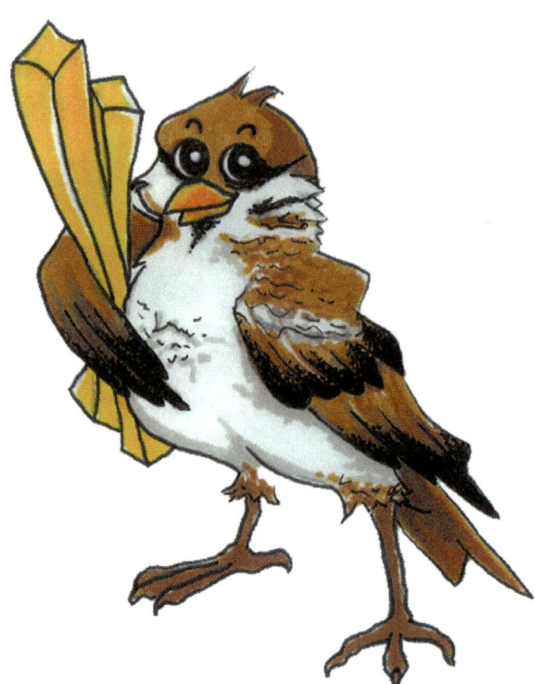

"I was looking to see if the children were down there eating some food," said Freddy.

"What kind of food?" Jeanie asked curiously.

"Real yummy food," replied Freddy.

"Is it dangerous to get that food?" asked Robby.

"No, not at all. The humans really like us. They give us food, and they laugh and say we're cute."

"Really?" chirped Alfie. "This sounds interesting."

"Let's go check out those humans," squealed Jeanie.

Freddy pointed out some brightly dressed boys and girls who sat at the tables laughing and talking while sipping on delicious pop and munching on long, crispy french fries.

"Oh, look. I see some children now," said Freddy.

Robby was growing impatient. "Well, let's go!" he called.

"Oh, what is that red stuff?" cried Jeanie. "That looks awful." She puffed out her feathers to show her disgust.

Freddy laughed. "Ha, ha. That's really tasty! The children call it ketchup."

Jeanie giggled. "Ketchup, that's a funny word."

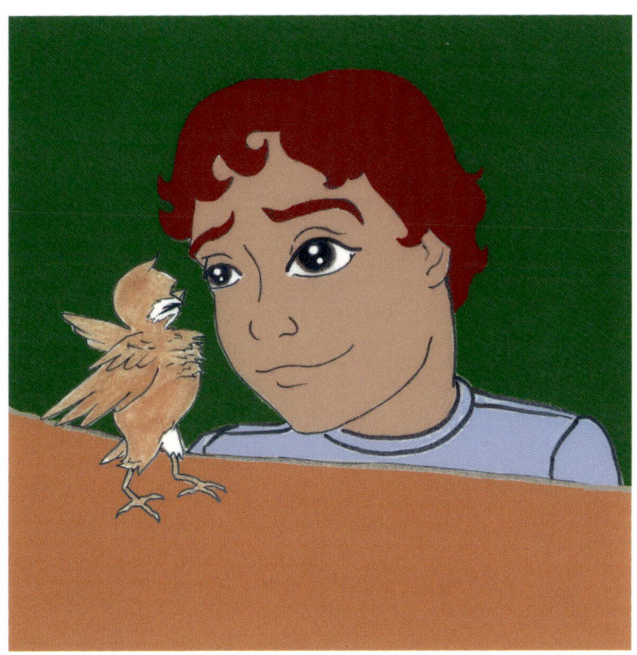

Robby had already flown over to the tables, boldly landing right in the middle of the table where the children were eating. One of the boys, dressed in blue shorts and a T-shirt, pushed back a shock of dark brown hair. With his brown eyes wide with curiosity and interest, the young boy leaned forward to look at Robby. Robby ruffled his feathers and bravely stared back. He tried to look like a big, mean bird!

Robby was a bit scared but tried to be courageous. Far away, from the rooftop, the children looked small, but this close, they were really big!

Slowly, the boy picked up a french fry and held it up to Robby. The french fry shimmered in the bright sunlight as a drop of fat dripped to the table. Timidly, Robby leaned forward and stretched his neck to reach the french fry. Cautiously he took a nibble and swiftly flew off, to the safety of the rooftop.

"Wow, this is good!" yelled Robby as he smacked his small beak. "This is sooooo yummy!"

Knowingly, Freddy nodded. "Yup, I know. They are very good, huh?"

"I want more! More!" squealed Robby as he flew away.

Robby was so excited about the french fries that he did not watch where he was flying. He swooped down towards the table and started to land. Poor Robby did not see he was going too fast, and he landed on the table with a big thump. His little wings spread out like an eagle.

He skidded across the greasy tabletop and ended up headfirst in a blob of ketchup. His head was covered with ketchup. Shocked, he tried to shake off the red sauce, but it was too sticky. One at a time, he opened his eyes and peered through the ketchup to see where the other french fries were.

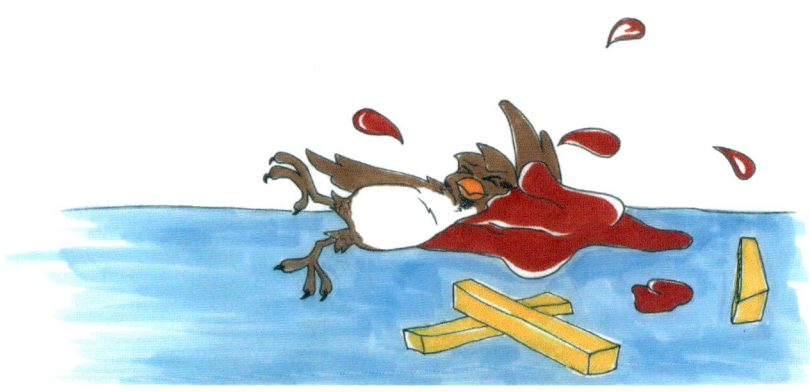

The children had stopped talking and were staring at the little bird covered with ketchup. A little girl with bright red curls, blue eyes, and freckles burst out laughing.

She pointed at Robby. "Look, look! What a funny bird!"

Poor Robby! He just wanted another french fry. He shook himself, and without looking at the children, he walked over to a paper plate where the french fries were spread out. Robby picked one up in his beak and quickly flew away to enjoy his meal.

Chapter 4

Freddy's Nightmare

In the darkness, Freddy snugly huddled in his Styrofoam and paper nest, against the warm bricks of the chimney. In the distance, he could hear the steady hum of the cars driving along the highway with their lights flashing brightly as they slowed to steer through a curve. He squinted his eyes, and the lights looked like a long, sparkly necklace.

The day had been an exciting one. Freddy's friends had come to meet him, they all had met some friendly children, and Robby had tasted his first french fries. Freddy chuckled to himself when he remembered how Robby had skidded through the grease on the table and had landed headfirst in the ketchup. What a funny sight that was!

With a soft grunt, Freddy shifted his weight to get comfortable and scratched his belly, but could not reach his belly button. Puzzled, he looked down and saw a large, round belly sticking out. Still bewildered, he scratched his head and looked at his belly. He hadn't noticed he couldn't reach his belly button before! His belly hadn't been that big…or had it?

Come to think of it, he soon realized he was no longer comfortable in his little nest—not like a few weeks ago, when he had first built it. Could it have shrunk in the rain? Otherwise, maybe Alfie, Jeanie, and Robby had played a trick on him and changed the size of his nest.

"Maybe… maybe…" mumbled Freddy. With a sigh, he shifted his weight one more time to get comfortable. Then his little black head nodded and his eyes slowly closed as he drifted into a deep, deep sleep.

As he slept, Freddy's eyes sometimes fluttered and he flapped his wings while moaning softly. Freddy was having a very bad dream…

It was a warm, humid day. The sky was a deep blue, and the sun shone cheerfully. Since no wind was blowing, the leaves of the trees lay heavy and limp on their branches.

Not feeling the heat, Jeanie danced around in the sky, enjoying herself. "Look at me!" she giggled. "I'm flying higher and higher! Wheeee! This is a lot of fun."

With his little yellow beak thrown open, Robby sat on a branch panting. It was a warm day and he did not like it. He was tired and listlessly watched Jeanie diving and twirling in the sky, when all of a sudden he noticed a big hawk coming her way.

"Hey, watch out for the hawk!" screeched Robby. "He's coming to eat you!"

"Robby, come up here; it is wonderful!" squealed Jeanie. "You can see everything! Boats are sailing on the lake, far, far away! And, the yummy bugs are way up here today!"

"No! You come down here! Watch out for the hawk! He's coming!" yelled Alfie, who was perched next to Robby on the branch in the nearby tree.

Jeanie laughed. "Oh, you boys are so scared!" "Look at me! Weeee!"

Jeanie was not aware of the danger. The hawk was diving right at her as she danced through the air, giggling and catching a few tasty insects.

Freddy was watching from his nest and tried to get to the edge of the roof to fly off and warn Jeanie about the approaching hawk. He slowly waddled to the edge and flapped his wings. And...nothing. He could not get himself into the air. He tried again, desperate to help his little friend. He flapped his wings but nothing happened. The hawk was coming closer and closer.

Freddy started to yell, trying to get the hawk away from Jeanie. "Hey, hawk, over here! Over here! Come get ME!"

Jeanie noticed a shadow hovering over her and looked up. She realized it was the hawk and knew she was in danger.

"Oh, please, please help me!" wailed Jeanie as she scrambled to get out of the hawk's way.

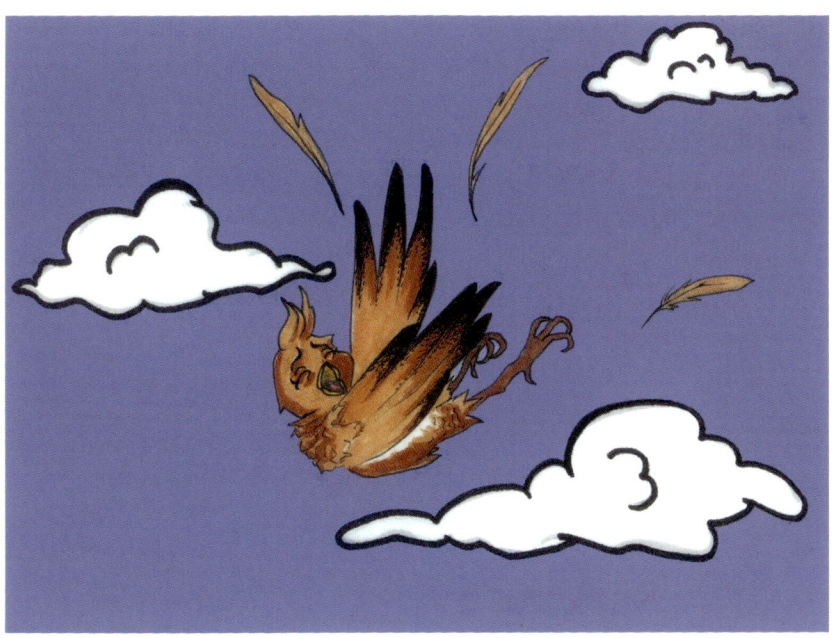

Freddy's screams had distracted and confused the hawk. The hawk looked up and bumped into Jeanie, who went tumbling through the sky. In an instant, the hawk shook his head and directed his attention to Freddy.

Hmm, this is a nice chubby one, thought the hawk. Nice to eat!

With a gulp, Freddy understood he was in trouble. He flapped his wings to fly away but could not get off the ground. He flapped and flapped.

He saw the hawk's beady eyes and thought he looked

hungry. The hawk came closer and closer, and Freddy kept flapping his wings. The hawk threw out his large talons and...

Freddy awakened with a start, his little heart pounding in his chest. His tiny yellow beak was damp with sweat. His feathers were damp, too. He shivered and looked around to see where the scary hawk was. He couldn't see the hawk anywhere. Freddy sighed and groaned in relief.

Dawn had arrived, and Freddy saw his three friends sleeping peacefully with their parents in their warm nests. Dewdrops hung from the branches and spiderwebs. The sun started to peek out from the horizon, making the lake a deep orange.

Phew, that was a horrible nightmare! thought Freddy, and he shivered again. He sat for a few minutes to calm down.

Then he remembered that he could not fly in his nightmare. Hoping that wasn't true, Freddy got up from his nest and tried to flap his wings. He was curious to see if he could get off the ground. He flapped and flapped. Nothing! Freddy couldn't fly! Feeling confused, he tried again. He could flap his wings, but he did not leave the ground.

Freddy was shocked. He stared down at his round belly and frowned. What was the problem? This had never happened to him before. His wings worked fine, but they were not strong enough to carry him up into the air because his belly was too big.

What had happened? He remembered what his mother had told him. She had said, "Freddy, you cannot eat so many french fries. That's human food, and not good for you."

Freddy had laughed and told his mother, "It's okay, Mama. Don't worry."

He realized what had happened. He had not listened to his mother and had eaten too many french fries. Now he could not fly.

"Oh, no! This is awful!" cried Freddy.

He wished he had listened to his mother and had gone to play with his friends instead of eating the french fries. Sitting in his nest, he had watched as his friends were having fun, catching bugs and other insects. After that they would visit Tommy, the tomcat.

"Humph, french fries are much tastier than those silly bugs we always eat," muttered Freddy.

"I'm sure it wasn't the french fries! It couldn't be the french fries!"

Freddy sighed. He knew he had eaten a lot of fries. His mother had told him too many were not good for you. He had eaten far too many of them, and now he was a chubby bird.

Realizing he was overweight, Freddy hung his head, slumped his shoulders, and waddled back to his nest. With a few grunts and groans, Freddy lowered himself into it. He tried to get comfortable but couldn't. He realized the rain had not shrunk his nest—he had outgrown it!

Slowly a single tear slid down his plump cheek, then one more, and then another. He started sobbing and sobbing. His little shoulders shook as he wept.

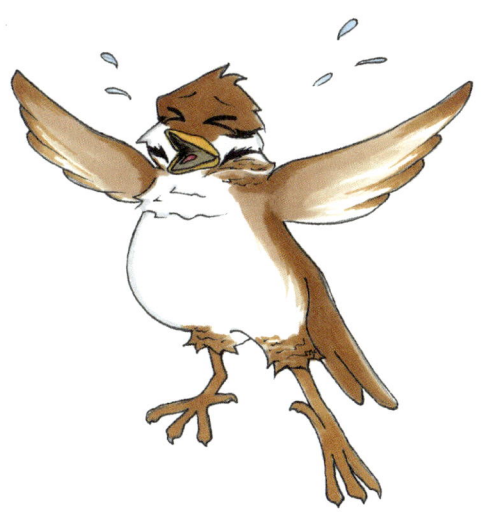

Chapter 5

Freddy Can't Fly

The sun chased away the soft morning mist that lay on the surface of the lake as a protective blanket. The dewdrops from the branches and spiderwebs had disappeared. A few regal swans swam by serenely as they headed towards the middle of the lake.

Alfie, Jeanie, and Robby woke up, stretched, yawned, and stretched again.

They were eager to start their day and hoped it would be filled with lots of fun and adventure.

"What do you want to do today?" asked Jeanie, hopping from one foot to the other.

Alfie shrugged. "I don't know. Maybe we can go visit Tommy. We can try to drink from his water bowl again. Last time was so thrilling!"

"Let's get some more french fries!" chirped Robby.

"That's a great idea!" squealed Jeanie, "but I want to show I can drink from Tommy's water bowl. Last time, I didn't get a chance because of Robby. Right, Robby?"

Robby grinned sheepishly. "Yeah, right."

The three friends flew off in the direction of the lake. Laughing and shrieking, they chased each other through the air, flying up, and up, and up, and then diving down again.

"Let's see if Freddy is awake yet!" called out Alfie.

"Yes, let's go joke with him!" chirped Robby.

Flapping her wings, Jeanie looked over to the chimney where Freddy had made his nest. She could see the colorful paper in Freddy's nest perched between the chimney and the satellite dish. She spotted Freddy and he appeared to be awake. But something was wrong. He was huddled in his nest and looked miserable.

Let's go cheer up Freddy," giggled Jeanie. "He doesn't look happy. I wonder what's wrong."

Alfie, Robby, and Jeanie turned and flew towards the rooftop where Freddy lived. Side by side, the three friends stood in front of Freddy's nest tilting their heads from side to side as they looked at Freddy curiously. Freddy looked sad and forlorn. He didn't even notice his friends had arrived. Why was Freddy so sad? Alfie, Robby, and Jeanie looked at each other and shrugged their feathered shoulders.

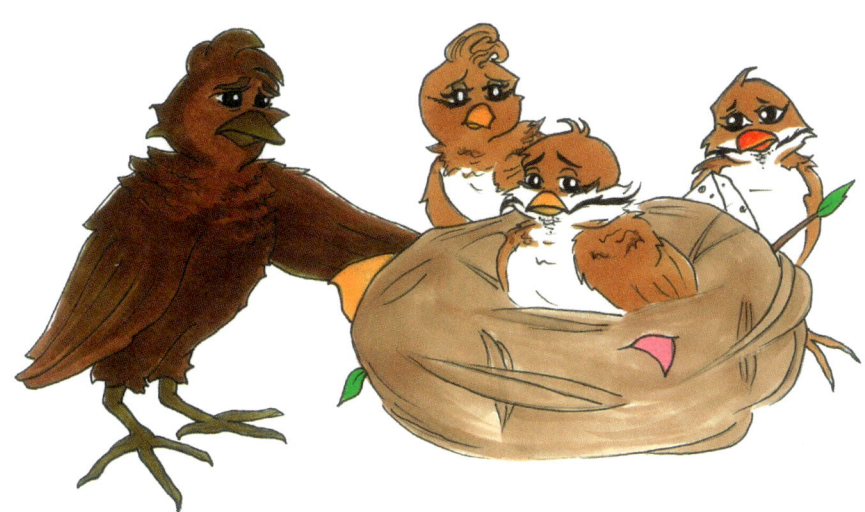

"Hey, Freddy...Freddy," murmured Jeanie. "Why are you so sad?"

"Yeah, Freddy, why are you crying?" asked Alfie.

Robby joined in worriedly. "Yeah, Freddy, why are you sad?"

"Well…well…" stuttered Freddy, "I had a bad dream and a hawk nearly ate Jeanie."

"Ah, that was just a dream!" Alfie then tapped Jeanie on the shoulder.

"See. Jeanie is still here."

"I know!" wailed Freddy. "That isn't why I'm crying. I'm crying because, in my dream, I couldn't fly."

Jeanie giggled. "That's so, so silly!"

"Birds can always fly," chirped Robby.

"It was just a dream," replied Alfie, patting Freddy on the back.

"No, no it's true. I can't fly!" moaned Freddy. "Look!" He then pushed himself up, waddled to the edge of the rooftop, and demonstrated his inability to fly. He flapped his wings to show his friends he couldn't get off of the roof. Sure enough, he was not able to fly away.

Alfie, Robby, and Jeanie gasped in surprise—a sparrow that couldn't fly; they didn't know what to think.

"See?" said Freddy with a deep sigh. "I can't fly!"

"Hmmm," muttered Alfie, "Hmmm." This matter was a serious one, and he sank down on the rooftop to think. Robby sat down beside him and propped his fist under his chin.

"But why Freddy? Why can't you fly?" asked Jeanie curiously.

"Because, because…oh…I…I ate too many french fries!" cried Freddy. "My mother told me they weren't good for me. And I was too lazy to play with you. I always wanted to nap or just sit and look around. Take a look at my plump belly."

With a sad, sad sigh, Freddy pointed to his round belly. Jeanie's eyes grew bigger. Now she understood why Freddy could not fly. Turning to Alfie, she said, "Alfie, we need to help Freddy. He needs to fly again. How can we help him?"

"Hmmm," mumbled Alfie. "Hmmm." He scratched his head. "Hmmmm," he said for the third time.

"Is that all you can say?" yelled Jeanie impatiently. She hopped up and down. "We need to help Freddy! Freddy needs our help!"

The four little friends huddled together in the early light of dawn, each deep in thought.

"I've got it! I've got it!" shouted Alfie enthusiastically. He jumped up and hopped from one foot to the other.

"What?!" cried Freddy, Jeanie, and Robby in chorus.

"Well," said Alfie as he ruffled his feathers and puffed out his chest. "Do you remember when we were flying over the park a few weeks ago?"

"Uh-huh," said Jeanie. "So what!"

"Do you remember we were teasing a human who was running?" asked Alfie.

"That was so much fun!" snickered Robby while remembering.

"And do you remember how we made him run faster when we began to dive towards him?" continued Alfie.

Jeanie crossed her wings and sniffed. "So, you want to tease Freddy and dive towards him? That's not nice, Alfie! We want to help him, not tease him!"

"No, no. You don't get it," cried Alfie impatiently. "Freddy needs to run!"

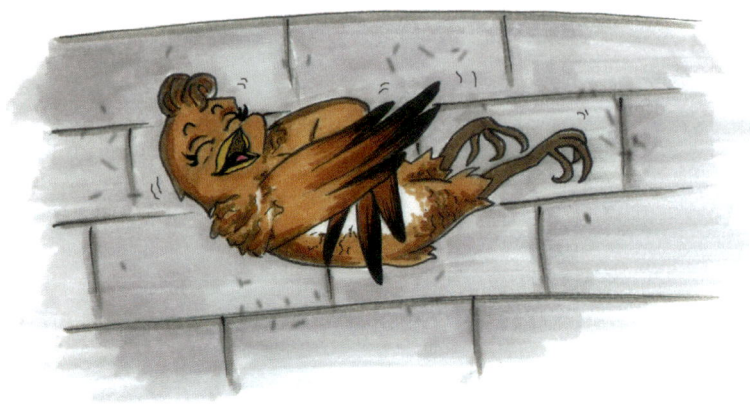

"Run?" squealed Jeanie. She toppled over and rolled on the rooftop, laughing and holding her own feathered belly. "Run? Have you ever heard of a bird that runs? He needs to fly!"

"I know. I know," shouted Alfie, annoyed, "but he needs to start with a little bit of exercise. He needs to lose his chubby belly."

"Uh-huh," chimed Jeanie, "and he has to stop eating those french fries. I heard my mother talking to Robby's mom, and they said that too many french fries aren't good for us, just as eating too many fries is not good for humans. But they do taste good!"

"Yeah, they are really good! cried Robby.

"Well, we need to help Freddy, so we can all stop getting the french fries and encourage Freddy to run," said Alfie.

Poor Freddy! He did not like the idea of running. He wanted to fly again and continue to eat that yummy food. Freddy groaned, "No, no." He could not give up his favorite food—those yellow sticks known as french fries. He smacked his beak just thinking about them.

"Oh, this is so horrible," sobbed Freddy. Robby hopped over to Freddy and put his wing around his friend's chunky shoulders.

Alfie was determined to help Freddy succeed. "Don't you worry," said Alfie. We're going to help you fly again."

Jeanie nodded. "Yes. We'll help you, for sure."

Chapter 6

Working Hard

The day had been very busy, and Freddy was tuckered out from all that had happened. His friends had left a while ago, and the rooftop had grown quiet.

Freddy snuggled into his warm nest, cuddling up to the squeaky, white Styrofoam. He watched as the moon climbed higher and higher into the sky. The silvery beams glowed gently on the water and made it sparkle. He heard a lonely bird cry out in the distance. A few geese floated by quietly on the way to their nests, getting ready to sleep. A soft breeze rustled the leaves of the trees as Freddy got ready to sleep. He heard a few ducklings calling for their mother as the family members made their way to their own nest for a good night's sleep. He heard the steady hum of cars driving along the highway. Listening to all the familiar noises of the night, Freddy settled into his nest and groaned. Oh, he was so tired, but very happy.

Grinning, he fondly thought of Alfie, Jeanie, and Robby. They were such good friends. They wanted to help him lose his big belly and were planning to work hard to help him do so.

The next morning, Alfie, Jeanie, and Robby were up early and busy preparing the area for Freddy to exercise. Alfie worked hard to supervise the preparations on part of the rooftop. All day Alfie bossed everyone around. He directed Jeanie and Robby to collect sticks, twigs, berries, and acorns. He pointed out to Freddy where to put them.

Huffing and puffing, Freddy sat on the ground. He had worked hard to help Alfie with the preparation of his exercise area.

"Hey, Alfie, is this good?" asked Robby as he dropped a few berries onto a pile and wiped his brow.

"Yup!" called Alfie. "Get some more!"

"You're too bossy," sniffed Jeanie. "Why don't you collect those twigs and things?" She flew off to get more.

"Because," yelled Alfie, "I'm the boss."
The rooftop was being transformed into a gym—a special gym for Freddy. Near the satellite dish was a heap of acorns.

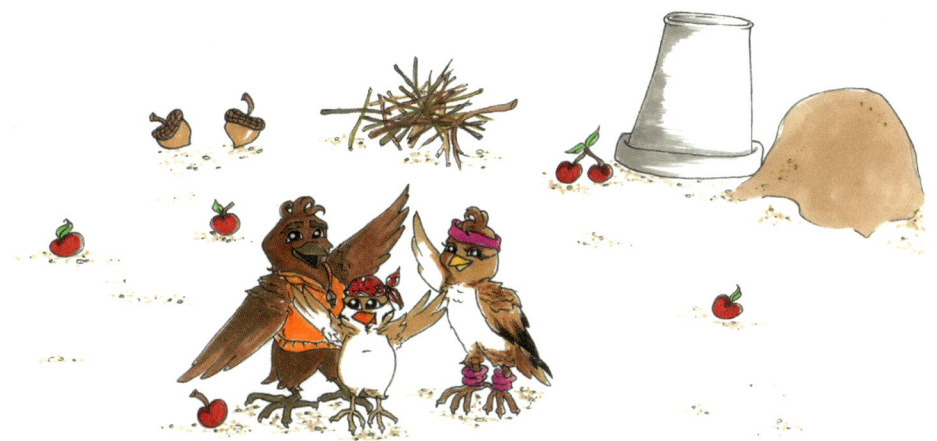

On the other side, Robby had piled up berries. Jeanie had scattered the twigs all around.

The day had been busy for Freddy's three friends. Alfie, Jeanie, and Robby were sitting on a branch in a tree nearby the rooftop. They saw Freddy snuggled up into his nest.

Jeanie sighed. "I hope Freddy will like the track. Do you think he will?"

"Mmmmm, I think so!" mumbled Alfie. "I think so."

"I know he will!" said Robby as he let out a yawn. "Now let's go to sleep."

The three friends flew to their parents' nests and went to sleep.

Chapter 7

Time to Exercise!

"Hey, get up Freddy!" shouted Alfie. "Get up!"

Freddy groaned, stretched his wings, turned around, and cuddled into his soft, warm nest.

"Freddy, you've got to get up! It's time to exercise. Today is the big day!" chirped Jeanie as she jumped up and down.

Exercise? thought Freddy. He sighed while burrowing his tiny head deeper into the warmth of his nest.

"Hey, Freddy. Freddy, you've got to get up," called Robby as he tugged at Freddy's wing. "C'mon. The sun is coming up really soon!"

With all the noise his friends were making, Freddy couldn't sleep any longer. He groaned, slowly rolled over, stretched his wings, and gingerly opened one eye.

In front of him stood his three best friends, wide-awake and full of energy. Alfie, dressed in an orange jogging suit, was jumping from one foot to the other; Jeanie wore a pink

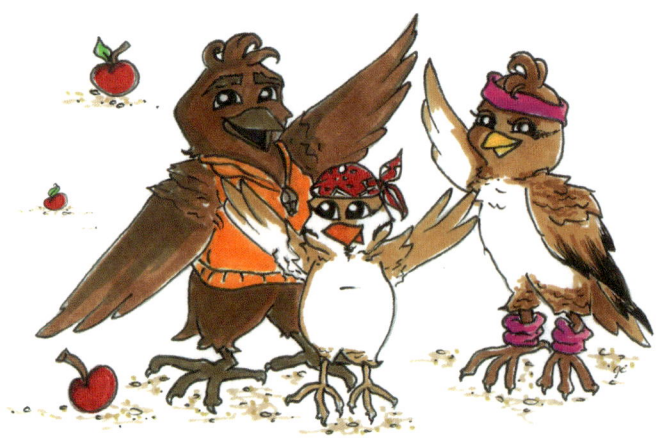

headband and leg-warmers to match. Impatiently she tilted her head from side to side. Robby had a red bandana wrapped around his little head and was jumping up and down, as well.

"Okay, okay. I'm ready," said Freddy as he slowly stood up in front of his friends. Yawning, he stretched his wings one more time and scratched his belly.

Jeanie giggled. "Look at your head. Your feathers are all sticking up. That is sooo funny!"

Quickly Freddy tried to push the feathers on his head down, but they popped up again. Jeanie giggled; he looked very funny.

"Okay. Put this on your head," said Alfie, holding out a blue headband. "We've got to get started!"

The four friends hopped over to the track that Alfie, Jeanie, and Robby had helped build. As the sun started to peak from the horizon, Freddy stood still and looked around at what his friends had set up for him. He saw a bunch of twigs stacked to one side. Beside the twigs Freddy saw berries scattered around the track. A few acorns were placed side by side. A mound of sand was piled to one side, and to the left of the sand Freddy saw an old Styrofoam cup, which was placed upside down.

Curiously, Freddy looked at Alfie. "What's all this for?"

Alfie pointed to the track proudly. "This is your training track."

Freddy stared at it with big eyes. Alfie started to explain what Freddy needed to do.

"First, you run to the pile of twigs. You need to pick up each twig, bring it back to us, and pile them all up here." Alfie pointed to the start line. "After that, you go to the berries. Those you need to pile up near the satellite dish." Alfie pointed in the opposite direction. "Then, you go to the acorns. You need to lift them over your head--as many as you can--and place them in a neat row beside the berries. And then, you need to run up and down the pile of sand twice. After that, you go to the cup and climb on top of it, jump down, and run back..."

Robby interrupted as he eagerly jumped up and down. "Doesn't that look like fun, Freddy? Doesn't it!"

But, as Freddy listened to Alfie's and Robby's directions, his eyes grew bigger and bigger.

"I can't do that!" wailed Freddy. "I want to go back to bed!" He pulled off his blue bandana and started to walk back to his comfortable nest.

Jeanie jumped right in front of him, her wings crossed over her tiny chest. With a frown on her face, she jeered, "Well, Freddy, I thought so. I told Alfie you couldn't do it. I knew you only wanted to sleep and eat and that you would not try it!" She stomped her foot.

Robby spoke up, defending his friend. "Jeanie, that isn't nice to say, you know."

"Well, it's true," said Jeanie with a sneer. "Freddy just wants to sleep and eat and do nothing!"

"I do not," replied Freddy, stomping his leg.

"Yes you do! Yes you do!" taunted Jeanie as she adjusted her leg warmers that had slipped down.

Freddy was very angry with Jeanie. "I do not!" he yelled.

Robby turned to his friend. "Show her, Freddy! You show her!"

Freddy sighed and hung his little head. Slowly he tied his

bandana around his head, turned, and waddled to the start of the track.

"You can do it, Freddy," encouraged Alfie. "Show Jeanie she's wrong!"

With a moan and a groan, Freddy started to run. He slowly trotted towards the pile of twigs, bent over, grumbled, and picked one up. Pausing to catch his breath, he shifted the twig in his arms and jogged back to where his friends stood waiting. He dropped the twig at their feet.

Alfie cheered. "Good for you. Go get the next one."

Feeling a bit encouraged and wanting to show Jeanie she was wrong, Freddy went to get the next twig, and the next one, and the next one after that. After a few times back and forth, Freddy finally dropped the last twig in the sand in front of his friends.

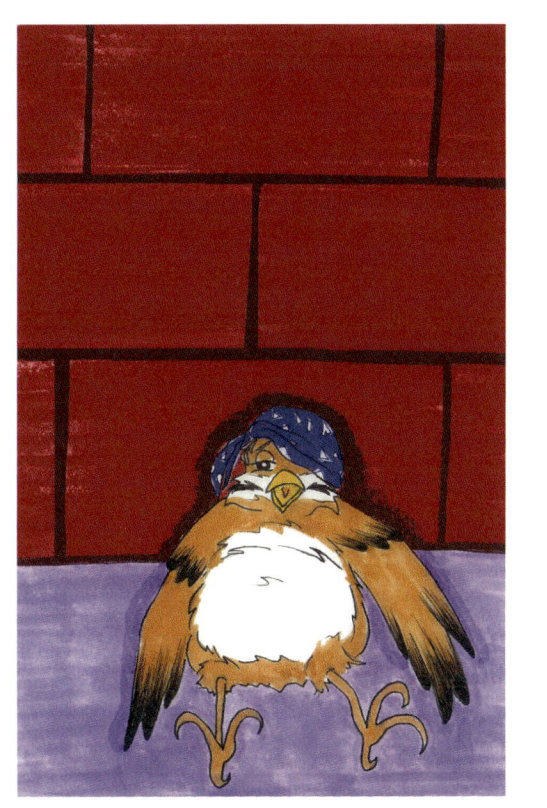

Huffing and puffing, he leaned against the chimney trying to catch his breath. His tiny chest was heaving, and his little beak opened wide to get more air. His bandana had slipped to one side, covering his eye.

"Here. Sip this. You must be thirsty," said Alfie as he held up a plastic lid, which he had found near the garbage bin. It held rainwater for Freddy, and Freddy gratefully took a sip but immediately spit it out.

"Yuck." Freddy didn't like it at all. "What is that?"

Surprised, Alfie looked at Freddy and said, "Water. It's good for you."

Freddy was not happy. "Yuck," he repeated, "I want my brown water! You know, the one that the children drink." Freddy stomped his foot.

"But Freddy, water is much better for you than pop," said Jeanie. Trying to decide what to do, she scratched her head and then offered a suggestion. "Maybe we can put some berries in the water. That might taste better," she said..

"Yeah, Freddy. Try that," chirped Robby. "You have to try!"

Freddy hesitated. "Well…well, okay. I'll try that." He realized his friends were trying to help him, and he was not being very nice to them.

Jeanie brought him a little bit of water with some of the berry juice squeezed into it. Gingerly, Freddy took a sip, and another one.

Freddy grinned. "This tastes good. I like this drink," he said as he pushed his bandana back onto his head. He was starting to feel better.

Chapter 8

Freddy Has a Rest

"You know, Freddy, you've worked very hard today. I think you deserve a rest. Robby and Jeanie and I are going to watch the ducklings and maybe spy on some humans in the park," said Alfie.

Freddy sighed. "Okay. I am tired." He then calmly wandered over to his nest and lay down.

Jeanie flew off and circled around them. "Hey, look over there! I see a few fat bugs. I'm really hungry."

"Wait for me, Jeanie. Wait for me," called Robby.

"Hey, slowpoke, come catch me if you can," said Jeanie with a giggle as she danced in the air.

Alfie looked at Freddy. He was concerned about his friend. "Are you okay, Freddy?"

"Sure," replied Freddy. "I'm really tired though. I'm going to take a nap."

"Okay," called Alfie as he pushed up the sleeves of his orange jumpsuit. "If you need company, just call for us." And off he went, to catch up with his friends.

With a sigh, Freddy settled into his nest to relax. He could feel his little muscles aching--proof that he had worked hard today. He grinned.

As the sun set and its yellow and orange rays reflected over the water, all of the other animals were getting ready for the night. Freddy could hear the mother ducks and geese call for their children. A light wind blew and it swirled around, playing with the leaves.

Freddy sat quietly, thinking about his adventures today. He looked around and saw the twigs, berries, and acorns scattered around the rooftop. He was so tired, but satisfied with what he had achieved. He had carried heavy twigs, berries, and acorns. He had run up and down the sand mound, and he had jumped up and down from the Styrofoam cup. The day had been fun, but now Freddy was worn out.

He watched his friends frolicking in the air before they, too, went to sleep. They were having fun, but Freddy felt very lonely. He wanted to play with his friends. Pulling off his bandana, he threw it into the air. It landed on top of the satellite dish.

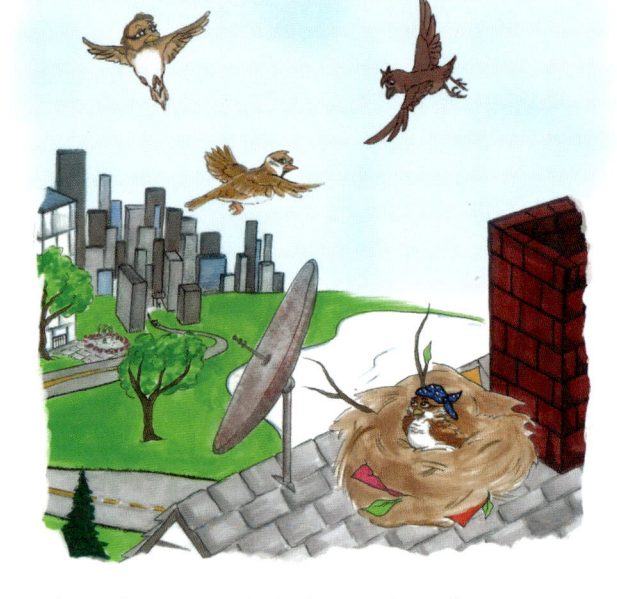

"I wish I could go with them," murmured Freddy as a lonely tear slid down his face.

Freddy rubbed his face, wiping away the tears. "I need to be able to fly again! I need to exercise, so that I can fly, too."

Determined, Freddy promised himself he would work hard to be able to fly once again. Before long he drifted into a restless sleep. His little wings were twitching, and once in a while, he moaned.

Freddy was dreaming again. He was dreaming that he could fly.

Alfie, Robby, and Jeanie were sitting on a branch in a

treetop nearby. The sun shone brightly in the clear blue sky. Freddy's friends were calling him. He flapped his wings and off he went! He was soaring through the sky. Freddy looked all around him. He saw the blue sky with the fluffy white clouds floating by him. He saw the little ducklings squabbling with each other. He saw the shiny cars driving along the highway. Freddy felt free as he frolicked through the air.

"Whoo-hooo...I can fly! I can fly!" called out Freddy. "Whoo-hooo!"

Then he saw the children in their brightly colored T-shirts and shorts eating their french fries and drinking their pop.

French fries! thought Freddy. He was mesmerized and forgot to flap his wings. Freddy began to tumble through the sky.

Alfie, Robby, and Jeanie gasped. "Oh no!" They raced off to rescue poor Freddy. As they reached their friend, he recovered and started to flap his wings again. Freddy flapped and flapped, and with great effort, he started to fly higher and higher.

"Freddy, you gave us a scare!" called out Jeanie.

"Yeah, Freddy, that was scary," said Robby.

"You have to focus, Freddy," yelled Alfie. "You scared all of us."

Freddy grinned. "I know. I scared myself, too! That won't happen again!"

All four friends giggled.

Freddy woke up giggling and flapping his wings. He grinned. What a weird dream!

Chapter 9
The Hawk

A few weeks had passed. Freddy had worked hard to lose his big belly. Today, Freddy exercised on the rooftop, one more time. With his blue bandana wrapped tightly around his feathery head and his little eyes shining brightly, he jogged around the track. He grabbed the twigs, ran across the track, and piled them up against the satellite dish. Next, he gathered the berries and piled them up. He trotted towards the acorns and lifted them above his head many, many times and lined them up in a neat row. Then, Freddy scampered across the track towards the mound of sand and ran up and down. After that he dashed towards the Styrofoam, and with a leap, he jumped up onto the cup and then down.

"Yahoo!" yelled Alfie, Jeanie, and Robby in chorus. "Freddy, you did it! You did it!"

With his head held high, Freddy pranced around the rooftop. He pushed out his chest, and with a great big grin on his little face, he said, "Yup. Yup, I did it! I'm healthy again!"

"It's time for you to see if you can fly and get off this rooftop!" yelled Alfie, jumping up and down.

Jeanie was excited. "This is the moment!" she called out.

"Freddy, this is wonderful!" chirped Robby. "You're going to fly again!"

Freddy stopped and froze in his tracks. "You mean, fly... in the air!" His voice sounded a bit panicky.

Jeanie giggled. "Of course, silly. Birds fly in the air!"

Freddy had a distraught look in his little eyes. "But... but... I don't know. I don't know if I can!" he wailed. "Maybe we can try it tomorrow!"

"Nah, Freddy, do it now," said Robby with encouragement in his voice. He grabbed Freddy by the wing and nudged him to the edge of the rooftop.

Freddy dug his heels in, but Robby pushed and pushed. Soon, Alfie and Jeanie started to push, too. Taking his time, Freddy slowly walked towards the edge of the rooftop.

"Fly, Freddy, fly!" called Alfie, Jeanie, and Robby.

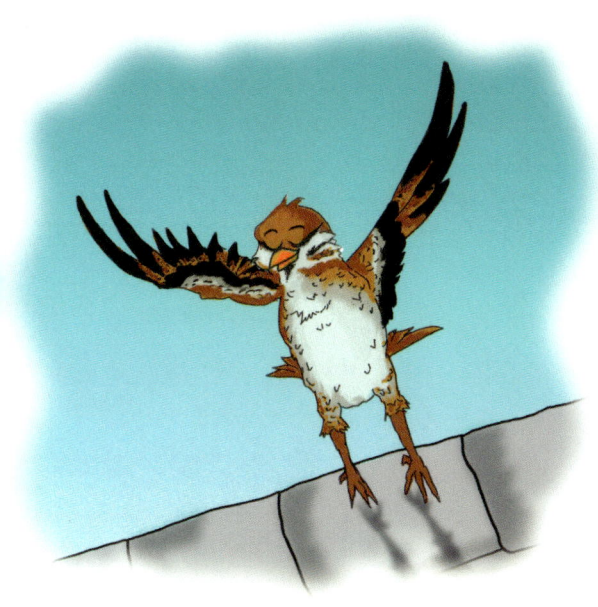

Freddy closed his eyes, and with a big, anxious sigh, he started to flap his wings. Up and up he went as his little friends cheered him on. Freddy slowly, carefully opened his eyes. He was flying! He flapped his wings again and again. Higher and higher, he climbed into the air. As he got higher up, Freddy felt braver and braver. He frolicked through the air, turning to see if his friends were watching.

"Whoo-hoo! This is great! I can fly! I can fly!" shouted Freddy as he flapped his wings.

"Oh, look. The juicy bugs are here. Let's go get some! And the baby ducks are following their mother! Let's go visit them, too. C'mon guys. Let's show off for the ducklings!"

Alfie, Jeanie, and Robby looked at each other, their little

faces beaming. With a high-five, they all took off and flew into the direction of Freddy, who was soaring through the air.

The three friends caught up with Freddy and planned a strategy for catching their meal of big, fat, juicy bugs. They flew higher and higher and then dove through the air towards the lake. They flew closer and closer to the lake, and then they turned and flew up and up again.

"This is so much fun!" said Jeanie as she flapped her wings and giggled.

"Yeah, this is sooooooo much fun!" squealed Robby as he soared through the air.

The little friends were having so much fun that they did not pay attention to their surroundings. Freddy looked up and, without any warning, saw a dark shadow coming towards them. It was the hawk—the hawk from his dream!

Freddy gasped and yelled, "Hey, look out! There's a hawk! Get out of the way! Oh, no!"

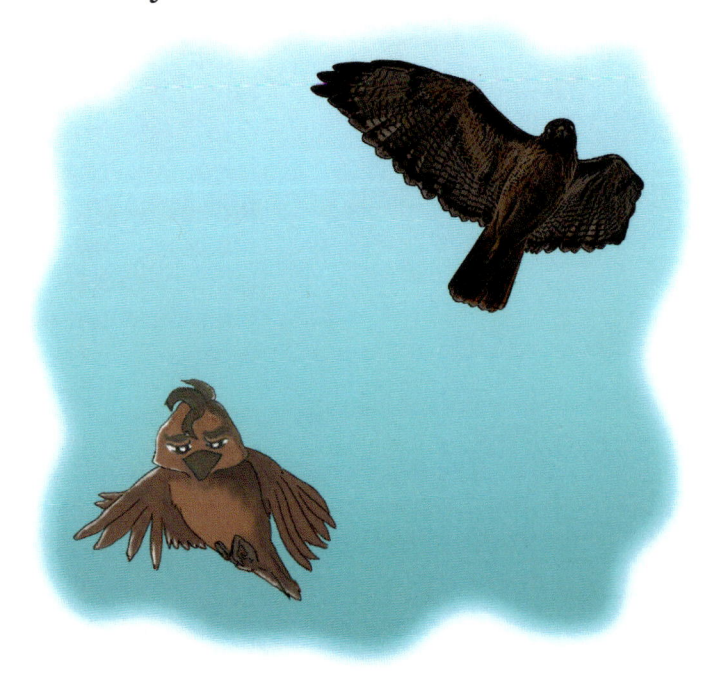

Alfie froze and then tumbled through the sky. He landed with a thump in Tommy's backyard, in between the thorn bushes. In an instant, Tommy woke up from his snooze and started to snoop around. He knew he had heard something but wasn't sure what.

Alfie lay dazed and confused but knew instinctively he needed to be very quiet. Tommy quietly roamed from one end of the yard to the other. He sensed there was something interesting in his garden.

Alfie jumped up, and in his haste, he hit his leg on a stone. "Ouch!" he yelled.

Tommy stopped and turned towards the area where he heard the noise. He got ready to pounce. Alfie quietly moved deeper into the thorn bush. When Tommy pounced, Alfie gasped. . .

Tommy landed in the thorn bush and got a face full of thorns. With an angry meow, he turned and walked away without even noticing Alfie.

Alfie sighed with relief. He was safe.

Meanwhile, the hawk had swooped towards Jeanie, and Jeanie flapped her wings with all her might. But the hawk was coming faster and faster.

"Oh no, Freddy. Please help me!" cried Jeanie.

Freddy started yelling. "Hey, hawk, come get ME! Come get ME!"

Distracted, the hawk turned his head towards Freddy and then plunged towards him.

With a worried look on his face, Freddy turned and flew towards the trees. His little wings were flapping and flapping. He could hardly breathe. Freddy was getting tired, but stopping would be too dangerous. The hawk was getting closer and closer. Freddy flew through the sky more swiftly.

Her eyes round with panic, Jeanie watched in horror while Freddy tried to get away from the hawk.

Then Freddy dove into a thick thorn bush. The hawk landed right in front of the bush, but was too big to squeeze inside. The thorns were sharp, but Freddy huddled deeper and deeper inside the bush. Disappointed, the hawk turned and flew away. He knew he could not get closer. Freddy was safe inside the bush.

Jeanie appeared and plopped down next to Freddy.

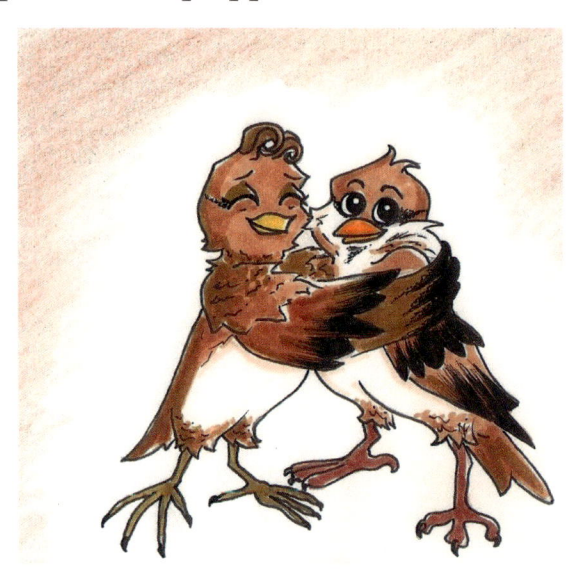

"Oh, Freddy, you saved my life!" She gave Freddy a great big hug. Wiggling to get free, Freddy said, "I'm glad you are alright, Jeanie. Now, let's go see if Alfie is okay."

"Alfie, where are you? Are you okay?" they yelled together.

"Yeah. Here I am. I'm okay. I was scared though! Tommy almost caught me! This has been a great adventure!"

Freddy and Jeanie giggled.

Chapter 10

Safe and Sound

"Hey," said Alfie, "where's Robby? Do you know where he is?"

Freddy and Jeanie looked at each other. They shrugged their shoulders and shook their heads.

"Oh no!" wailed Jeanie. "The hawk got him!"

"No!" yelled Alfie, determined to prove Jeanie wrong. "That can't be true. Let's go find him!"

Freddy nodded. "Let's go."

The three friends began to search for their friend, Robby. Alfie went to look near the bushes, and Freddy and Jeanie flew in the opposite direction towards the buildings.

"Robby," they called loudly. "Robby, where are you? Robby!"

After looking in the bushes, the trees, and near the tall buildings, they became more concerned. They had looked all over the place, but they couldn't find Robby anywhere.

Jeanie and Freddy flew to the treetops. Feeling discouraged, they perched on a branch. They sat quietly, in deep thought.

Then, in the distance, they heard someone giggling. They looked in the direction of the noise and saw Robby running around Freddy's exercise track. Robby was jumping up onto the Styrofoam cup and down again. He picked up an acorn and ran around the track, giggling some more.

"Robby!" called out Freddy. "Robby, are you having fun?"

With a big grin on his face, Robby stopped in his tracks and looked up. "Hey, guys, this is so much fun! Come join me!"

Freddy and Jeanie flew to the rooftop.

Then Alfie arrived. Out of breath, he shouted, "Robby! You're okay. Oh, I'm so happy! We were so worried about you!"

"There's nothing wrong with me. Why were you worried?" asked Robby curiously.

"Didn't you see the hawk?" asked Alfie.

"No. Where was the hawk?" asked Robby. He was getting excited. "Was there really a hawk?"

"Yeah!" shouted Jeanie, while she hugged Freddy.

"Freddy was soooo brave. The hawk had started to chase Alfie then me," chirped Jeanie, "but Freddy saved me."

"Wow!" gasped Robby. "That's really exciting."

"Yeah, and Alfie nearly got eaten by Tommy!" shrieked Freddy.

"Wow, Alfie! Wow, what an adventure!" cried Robby.

Robby scrunched up his face, hung his head, and shrugged his little shoulders. "I missed a great big adventure!" he cried.

The friends looked at each other and burst out laughing! They held their feathery bellies while they laughed and laughed.

"Well," said Freddy with a hiccup as he held his little belly, "today was a very busy day."

"Yeah, and you saved Jeanie's life!" said Alfie with a chuckle.

"And you nearly got eaten by Tommy," snickered Robby.

As the sun colored the sky a bright orange, the four little friends sat side by side. They were all in deep thought, remembering the day's adventures.

After a while, they became restless.

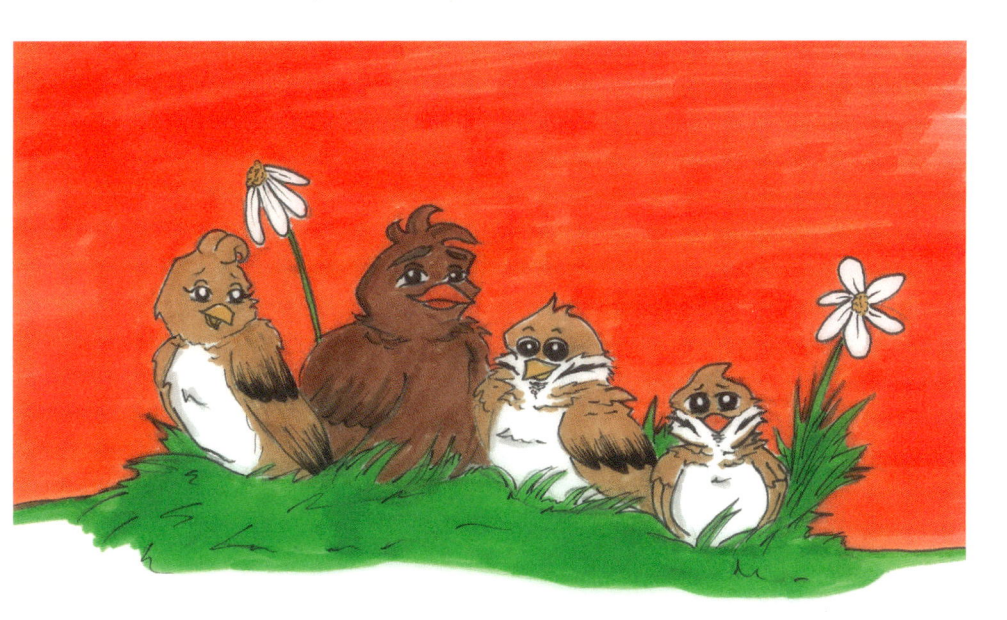

"Okay," called out Freddy, Alfie, and Jeanie in chorus, "let's do something."

"What do you want to do?" asked Alfie.

"We could visit the ducklings to see if they can fly yet," said Jeanie. "They're so cute when they're little, you know!"

Robby jumped up. "Or...or..." he said, "or we can see if Tommy is already sleeping."

"Sounds like fun!" called Freddy. "Let's go!"

The four friends flew away in the direction of the old, overgrown garden. As a day full of explorations finally came to an end, the four little friends were off looking for more new and exciting adventures.

The End

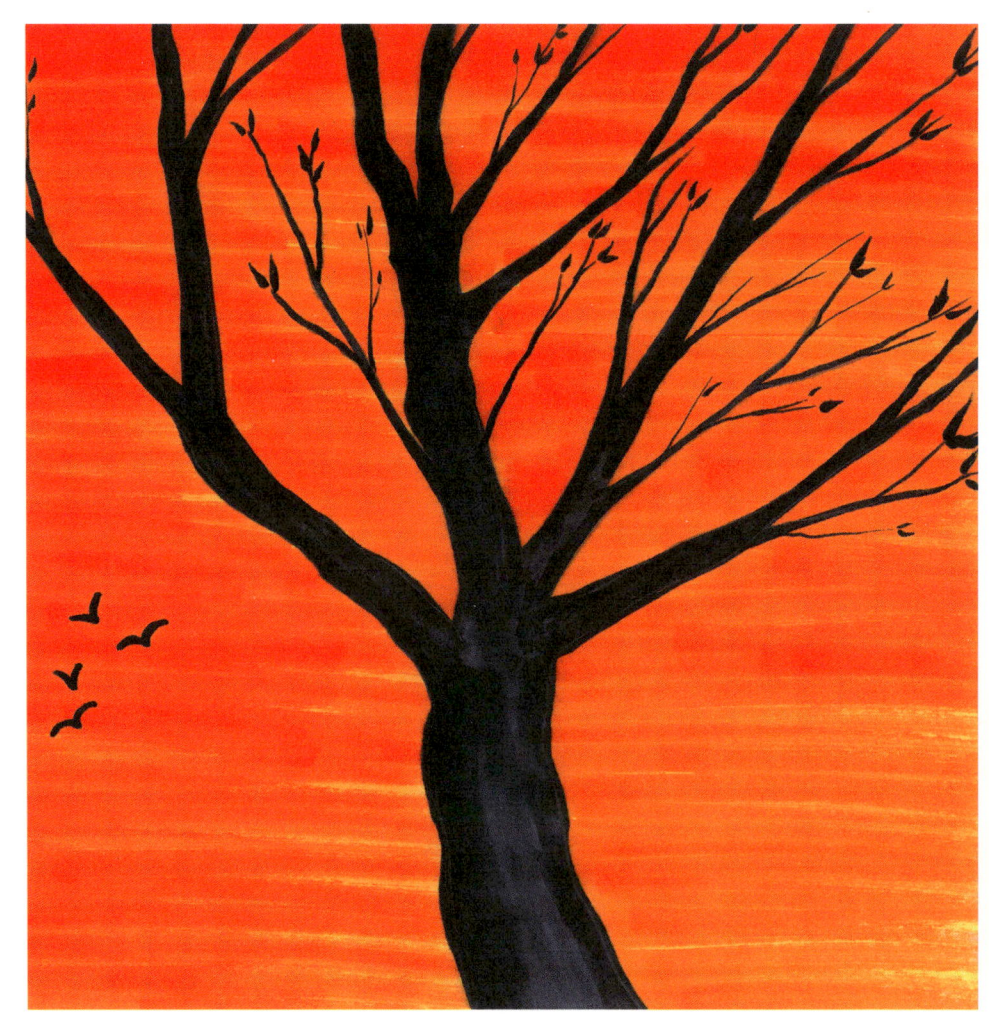

Testimonials

"Freddy's French Fries Fiasco" has it all! It is filled with great lessons from eating healthy, getting exercise, working hard towards your goals to the benefits of great friends who are there to support you when you need it most. It contains loads of adventures and keeps you riveted to the very end. A great book for parents to share with their children.

You are a very descriptive writer, DiDi making it easy to visualize the story, surroundings and the characters within.

P. Neill,
A Mom

> This book was a great read! It was funny and exciting. I especialy liked the part when Freddy fell into the ketchup

Tristen - Age 11

> It is a very absorbing book. I hope D.D. writes more books similar to this one because I love the way she describes the characters and settings.

Holly - Age 12

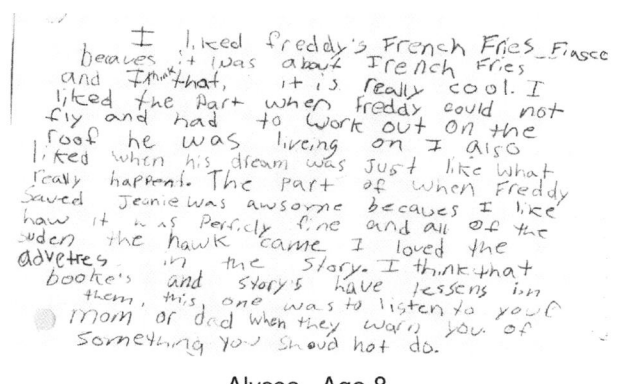

> I liked Freddy's French Fries Fiasco beaues it was about French Fries and I think that, it is really cool. I liked the part when freddy could not fly and had to work out on the roof he was liveing on I also liked when his dream was just like what realy happens. The part of when Freddy saved Jeanie was awsome becaues I like how it was perficly fine and all of the suden the hawk came I loved the advetres in the story. I think that booke's and story's have lessens in them, this one was to listen to your mom or dad when they warn you of something you should not do.

Alyssa - Age 8

CPSIA information can be obtained
at www.ICGtesting.com
Printed in the USA
LVIC040154080912
297856LV00002B